# MTHFR Diet

A Beginner's 2-Week Step-by-Step Guide to Managing MTHFR With Food, Includes Sample Recipes and a Meal Plan

## Disclaimer

By reading this disclaimer, you are accepting the terms of the disclaimer in full. If you disagree with this disclaimer, please do not read the guide.

All of the content within this guide is provided for informational and educational purposes only, and should not be accepted as independent medical or other professional advice. The author is not a doctor, physician, nurse, mental health provider, or registered nutritionist/dietician. Therefore, using and reading this guide does not establish any form of a physician-patient relationship.

Always consult with a physician or another qualified health provider with any issues or questions you might have regarding any sort of medical condition. Do not ever disregard any qualified professional medical advice or delay seeking that advice because of anything you have read in this guide. The information in this guide is not intended to be any sort of medical advice and should not be used in lieu of any medical advice by a licensed and qualified medical professional.

The information in this guide has been compiled from a variety of known sources. However, the author cannot attest to or guarantee the accuracy of each source and thus should not be held liable for any errors or omissions.

You acknowledge that the publisher of this guide will not be held liable for any loss or damage of any kind incurred as a result of this guide or the reliance on any information provided within this guide. You acknowledge and agree that you assume all risk and responsibility for any action you undertake in response to the information in this guide.

Using this guide does not guarantee any particular result (e.g., weight loss or a cure). By reading this guide, you acknowledge that there are no guarantees to any specific outcome or results you can expect.

All product names, diet plans, or names used in this guide are for identification purposes only and are the property of their respective owners. The use of these names does not imply endorsement. All other trademarks cited herein are the property of their respective owners.

Where applicable, this guide is not intended to be a substitute for the original work of this diet plan and is, at most, a supplement to the original work for this diet plan and never a direct substitute. This guide is a personal expression of the facts of that diet plan.

## Introduction

If you've been following the health and wellness scene at all in recent years, you've likely heard about MTHFR, even if you've never heard of the gene by that name. MTHFR is an abbreviation for methylenetetrahydrofolate reductase, an enzyme that plays a key role in converting folic acid into folinic acid and methionine, two chemicals used throughout the body. Folic acid is the synthetic form of folate, which is naturally found in foods.

While you can't control whether or not you inherited this gene mutation, it's still important to know about it. A lack of enzymes can be associated with various diseases and disorders such as cancer, vascular disease, and many more. If your MTHFR gene is defective, it can cause a variety of health problems.

A recent study published in the journal Nutrients found that people with MTHFR gene defects are more likely to have problems with obesity, insulin resistance, and fatty liver disease. The study authors suggest that people with MTHFR gene defects might benefit from a diet that is lower in sugar and saturated fat and higher in fiber.

Luckily, there are ways to work around these problems. One of the most popular methods is to follow a special MTHFR diet.

This diet focuses on eating foods that are high in folate and other nutrients that support MTHFR function. It also recommends avoiding foods that can interfere with folate absorption, such as sugar and saturated fat.

If you're interested in trying the MTHFR diet, this guide will show you how to get started. In this guide, you will discover...

- What the MTHFR diet is
- The benefits of following an MTHFR diet
- How to follow an MTHFR diet
- Sample recipes for the MTHFR diet

## What Exactly Is MTHFR?

MTHFR is an abbreviation for the enzyme methylenetetrahydrofolate reductase. Enzymes are proteins that act like little machines to speed up chemical reactions in your body.

MTHFR plays a key role in converting folic acid into folinic acid and methionine, two chemicals used throughout the body. They are used for important processes like creating the proteins your body needs and converting that leftover protein into energy. MTHFR mutations interfere with this process, making it difficult for the body to create these chemicals.

This can cause many health problems from birth defects to cancer to neurological damage. MTHFR mutations are linked to many chronic diseases and mental health issues. Approximately 30 to 40 percent of people have a form of the MTHFR gene mutation, but not everyone is affected the same way.

### *There are two main types: C677 and A1298*
The C677T mutation can lead to mood disorders and inflammation in the brain. The A1298C mutation can lead to depression and anxiety

A lack of the MTHFR enzyme can be associated with various diseases and disorders such as cancer, vascular disease, heart disease, some psychiatric disorders, miscarriages, infertility, and many more.

MTHFR mutations are common and are thought to affect an estimated 25 percent of Hispanics and up to 15 percent of Caucasians.

A recent study published in the journal Nutrients found that people with MTHFR gene defects are more likely to have problems with obesity, insulin resistance, and fatty liver disease.

MTHFR mutations can cause problems with detoxification and hormone metabolism, which means that the body cannot properly eliminate toxins and we may see increased levels of estrogen or heavy metals.

These mutations also interfere with neurotransmitters in the brain such as dopamine and serotonin, making it harder for us to regulate our moods. MTHFR mutations also contribute to cardiovascular disease so be especially careful if you have this mutation and are on birth control pills.

It is important to note that these problems do not occur for everyone who has an MTHFR mutation or a family history of heart issues, cancer, etc. This means that if someone  in your family has a history of these health problems, you should get tested to see if you have an MTHFR mutation.

### What typically causes MTHFR?
The mutant MTHFR gene is passed down through families. This mutation can be caused by a couple of different things.

• Genetics

First, some people have this mutation because it is actually coded in their DNA which means both of their parents have the mutation as well, so it is likely that they passed it on to you. An estimated 1 in 4 Caucasians have the MTHFR C677T mutation and 1 in 241 African Americans are carriers for this particular mutation. Some ethnicities are more affected than others. For example, only 18% of Ashkenazi Jews carry at least one copy of the MTHFR C677T mutation while 14% of African Americans do.

• Poor Diet and External Factors

Second, poor diet and environmental factors can make some people more likely to have MTHFR mutations. A lot of research shows that diets high in sugar increase oxidative stress which can lead to health problems like cardiovascular disease and cancer. Oxidative stress also damages DNA which increases the chance of genetic mutations.

Cigarette smoke is also an environmental factor that contributes to mutations especially with the MTHFR C677T mutation so be sure to avoid smoking if you have this mutation or are at risk of having it.

### *What are some symptoms?*

If your body does not produce enough methylfolate or methylcobalamin, you may start experiencing symptoms related to these chemicals. These include physical issues like constipation, headaches, irregular heart rate, gastrointestinal problems like gas and bloating, mental health problems like low mood or anxiety, neurological issues like seizures and tremors, skin pigmentation changes, lack of coordination, retarded growth in children (R) just to name a few.

Additionally, MTHFR mutations can interfere with the transportation of B vitamins throughout the body so levels may be lower than normal. Common deficiencies that come along with this mutation are Vitamin D3, folate/B9, and Vitamin B12. These vitamin deficiencies can also cause similar symptoms as having an MTHFR mutation alone.

## Getting Tested

Now that you are educated on how this mutation can affect the body, you may be asking yourself if it is necessary to get tested to find out whether or not you have an MTHFR mutation.

There are some health problems related to this mutation that you can check for yourself, but the only way to know if you have an MTHFR gene mutation is with a genetic test.

### *The genetic test for MTHFR mutations*

There are two types of genetic tests available for people who want to know if they have an MTHFR problem. The first test uses a blood sample to check the chromosomes. To get this test, you need to see a genetics specialist. If the blood test comes back positive for an MTHFR mutation, your doctor may refer you to a genetic counselor who can help you figure out if the mutation is causing health problems.

The second test uses saliva and looks at specific genes. With this type of testing, you collect your saliva sample at home and then send it off to be tested. You do not need a prescription or medical referral to take one of these tests. The downside is that they are often more expensive than the blood test, so many people opt for the less accurate blood test instead. The saliva test costs about US$200 while the blood test is only about half that price. It is also known that the saliva test is much more accurate than the blood test.

Here are some of the most common tests to check for an MTHFR mutation:
- DNA Genetic Testing by the genomics and biotechnology company 23andme
- Gene Variance Report by LiveWello
- Genetic Genie

## Managing MTHFR Through Diet

If you have tested positive for an MTHFR gene mutation, the next step is to learn how to manage this problem through diet and lifestyle. Currently, there is no medication to address this mutation. However, there are ways to manage your symptoms naturally.

The MTHFR diet is a special diet that can help with symptoms of MTHFR polymorphism. It is based on the principle that eating specific foods can help improve the function of your MTHFR gene. With this diet, you can help reduce the effects of low MTHFR enzyme activity in your body.

In general, your diet should be rich in nutrients and low in foods that contain folic acid because this nutrient may block the activity of your MTHFR enzyme. Focus on a healthy diet that is based on vegetables and fruits. You should increase the intake of veggies and fruits both in raw form and cooked form for best results.

### *Food to avoid on an MTHFR diet*

There are certain foods to be avoided when managing MTHFR symptoms through diet. These include:

• Caffeine inhibits the body's ability to process and absorb folic acid (vitamin B9). If you drink coffee, consider switching over to green tea or another caffeine-free herbal tea.

• Alcohol decreases the body's ability to absorb key nutrients necessary for methylation including folate, B12, and zinc. It also reduces levels of glutathione which is a powerful antioxidant that helps protect cells from damage caused by free radicals. If you choose to drink alcohol, limit consumption to two drinks a week or less.

• Processed sugar interferes with the body's ability to absorb vitamin B9 (folic acid). It also affects the absorption of zinc, which is needed for healthy immune function and proper metabolism.

• High-lycopene foods such as raw tomatoes and watermelon. While these foods are healthy, the lycopene found in them blocks the absorption of folic acid.

• Nuts block the body's ability to absorb folate.

• Processed foods should be avoided because they are often made with artificial ingredients—ingredients that can affect the body's ability to absorb and process vitamins.

• Iodine inhibits the body's ability to process and absorb folic acid. Seafood such as shrimp, lobster, and crab contains high amounts of iodine.

• High-mercury fish such as king mackerel, tuna steaks, swordfish, tilefish from the Gulf of Mexico, marlin, and orange roughy. Mercury is an extremely harmful toxin that can damage the nervous system.

• Processed meats often contain high levels of preservatives and other chemicals that interfere with the body's ability to absorb and process vitamins and minerals.

### Foods to eat on an MTHFR diet
As you can see, many foods need to be avoided when managing MTHFR symptoms through diet. Fortunately, there are also certain foods that you should include in the diet to help balance your MTHFR genes and improve your ability to process vitamins and minerals. These foods include:

• Leafy green vegetables are rich in folic acid, which is the natural form of the B vitamin folate. Folate counteracts homocysteine, a harmful chemical that can damage blood vessels and contribute to cardiovascular disease. Some examples of leafy green vegetables include spinach, avocado, and collard greens.

• Animal protein provides the body with key amino acids which are needed for proper methylation. These proteins also offer various nutritional benefits such as B vitamins, iron, and zinc.

• Legumes such as soybeans, lentils, kidney beans, pinto beans, black-eyed peas, chickpeas (garbanzo beans), green peas, and lima beans are all great choices because they contain high amounts of folate, an important nutrient in the methylation process.

• Herbs and spices are rich in magnesium. Some to consider adding to your diet include rosemary (B2), thyme, peppermint, garlic (vitamin C) parsley, basil cayenne pepper, and turmeric.

• Yogurt is a good source of probiotics that promote digestive health and balance the body's bacteria levels. It also contains vitamin B6.

Remember that in an MTHFR diet, aside from sticking to a balanced diet, the meals should contain the following nutrients: vitamins B2 (riboflavin), B6, B9 (folate), B12, C, D3, and E; along with betaine, choline, EPA/DHA, glutathione, n-acetyl-cysteine, and turmeric.

## How to Implement the MTHFR Diet

Now that you know what foods to eat and what foods to avoid, it is time to get started with this diet. The MTHFR diet can be challenging because it eliminates many of the foods that are normally included in a healthy diet. However, there are tips and tricks for sticking to the plan which will be discussed in-depth in this chapter.

### *Week 1*
During the first week, focus on understanding and studying more about the changes you have to do as you undergo the MTHFR diet. You may also start preparing yourself and your kitchen for this diet.

### • Plan on your diet menu
Take note of the foods you should eat and avoid. It's best to start with curating your menu for the duration of your diet program. Research the ingredients you will need for your menu. Doing so will also help you prepare your kitchen and your pantry with the ingredients you will need for your diet meals.

### • Discard foods you must avoid
Attempt to clear out the foods in your home that contain ingredients that must be avoided on your MTHFR diet. These include processed junk foods and foods high in preservatives. Grab a large garbage bag

and fill it with these foods so that you are not tempted to eat them.

## • Involve your family in your journey

One way to make sure you're able to start and finish this diet plan is to involve your family with your plan by being your source of support. They will be responsible for keeping you in check, particularly with the food you need to avoid. Make sure that they accompany you when you shop for the ingredients you will need for your meals.

## • Plan your grocery trip well

Start making a grocery list of the foods that you plan on eating. Plan out your meals for the week by looking online or at other cookbooks. Make sure that foods exclude all of the foods on the list of foods to avoid. If you need sample recipes, check out the later chapter in this guide for some quick and easy recipe ideas. This is also where your menu plan will come in handy.

Make sure that you avoid all the ingredients and foods that you don't need in your diet.

## • Make a food diary

It's advisable that you make a food diary of some sort, not only to help you keep track of the foods you must eat and avoid, but also to take note of the possible changes you may experience regularly throughout your diet plan.

This may also help you later in assessing how the program affected you and your overall health.

### • Begin with the diet transition

Another way to condition your mind and body with the diet plan is to slowly begin the transition to help your body adjust. You may ease into it by preparing one meal a day that fits the requirements for this diet program.

### • Create a weekly meal plan

Creating a weekly meal plan will help in making your diet journey more enjoyable and less tedious. This way, you won't have to worry about what to prepare because you already know what you must expect by following a meal plan.

The sample meal plan below is created to help you get an idea of how you can plan your diet program ahead of time. You probably prepared food that's good for more than one serving, so you may of course serve that again on your next meal. You can of course modify your meal plan according to what works best for you.

# Sample meal plan

|  | Breakfast | Lunch | Dinner |
|---|---|---|---|
| Monday | Grenade Salad | Chicken and Broccoli Casserole | Savory Chicken and Lentil Soup |
| Tuesday | Avocado and Quinoa Salad | Baked Salmon with Dill and Lemon | Lentil Soup |
| Wednesday | Greens Salad with Pesto Dressing | Sesame Chicken | Udon Salmon Soup |
| Thursday | Spinach and Watercress Salad | Grilled Lamb | Broccoli Soup |
| Friday | Quinoa Lentil Salad | Baked Chicken Breasts | Pepitas-Kale Soup |
| Saturday | Garlic Broccoli Salad | Ginger Chicken Stir Fry | Macrobiotic Bowl Medley |
| Sunday | Spinach Salad Mix | Instant Pot Bone Broth | Salmon Salad |

## *Week 2*

By the start of this second week, you should be equipped to start this diet program properly with your lists and recipes. This week will be an adjustment because you will have less food to choose from, but it will get easier as the week goes on.

- *Expect changes in your body*

You should expect some headaches or minor detox symptoms as your body adjusts to this new diet plan. Don't panic because this is normal and will pass in a few days.

## • *Take note of the changes you experience*

As your body adjusts to the effects of your diet changes, it is good to take note of these changes in your food diary. By the end of the two weeks, share the results with your physician so they can assess how the diet affected you and if you need to curate it for your future meal plans.

It's also advisable to be on the lookout for possible signs of additional symptoms due to the changes your body is experiencing. Take note of them in your food diary or contact your doctor if necessary.

## • *Add probiotics to your diet*

During this second week, stick with eating only the recommended types of food. In case the meals are not enough, you may add probiotics to your diet. Foods like yogurt contain probiotics which are beneficial for maintaining overall health and digestive system health specifically. Good sources of probiotics include Greek yogurt, organic soy yogurt, and regular unsweetened yogurt. You may have these as snacks.

## • *Always stay hydrated*

Make sure that you also stay hydrated by drinking plenty of water. Adding soups to your diet will also help in keeping you well-hydrated.

## • Consider taking supplements

Before adding this to your diet, make sure that you consult with your doctor first. Usually, taking supplements as a substitute for sources of nutrients in case you are unable to make meals with the needed nutrients is okay. Make sure that you heed the advice of your doctor regarding this.

## • Stick to eating organic and natural

In case you plan to eat out or want to try other meals, make sure that their ingredients follow what you need to consume. Strictly stick to eating natural and organic meals, also called 'clean foods.' This way, you can enjoy eating out without compromising your health.

By the end of the second week of your MTHFR diet program, it's best to consult with a doctor to find out how the initial dietary changes affected your body. This is also where your food diary will come in handy, especially if you included in your notes how each meal made you feel. From this, you may consider adjusting the ingredients or the quantity to better suit your needs and your lifestyle.

Because there isn't any cure for the MTHFR mutations, sticking to a healthier lifestyle is the best option for those who have this condition. Aside from that, you also benefit from these changes in the longer run.

**Sample Recipes**

## Grenade Salad

Ingredients:
- 4 cups arugula
- 1 large avocado
- 1/2 cup sliced fennel
- 1/2 cup sliced Anjou pears
- 1/4 cup pomegranate seeds

Instructions:
1. Mix all the ingredients except for the pomegranate seeds.
2. After mixing well, add the seeds. Mix again.
3. Serve with any type of desired dressing.

# Greens Salad with Pesto Dressing

Ingredients:
Salad:
- 1 head lettuce, chopped
- 1/4 bulb fennel
- 2 cucumbers
- avocado
- 1/4 cup basil leaves
- 1/8 cup dill
- black peppercorns
- 2 tbsp. lemon juice
- olive oil

Pesto Sauce:
- 1 lemon
- 1/2 cup arugula
- 1 cup olive oil

Instructions:
1. To make the pesto sauce, put all the ingredients in a food processor. Blend to smoothen.
2. Season with lemon juice, pepper, and salt. Transfer to a small bowl.
3. In a large salad bowl, toss the herbs and remaining vegetables.
4. Transfer pesto sauce to a small bowl, and serve with the salad.

5. In a pan, prepare the halloumi by frying until crunchy at the sides
6. Serve salad greens and pesto sauce.

# Garlic Broccoli Salad

Ingredients:
- 1 head broccoli, cut into florets
- 1 tsp. olive oil
- 1-1/2 tbsp. rice wine vinegar
- 1 tbsp. sesame oil
- 2 cloves garlic, minced
- 1 pinch cayenne pepper
- 3 tbsp. golden raisins

Instructions:
1. Fill water into a steamer. Bring to a boil.
2. Add broccoli. Cover. Steam until tender for about 3 minutes.
3. Rinse broccoli and set aside.
4. Heat olive oil in a skillet over medium heat.
5. Put in pine nuts. Stir fry for 1-2 minutes.
6. Remove from heat.
7. Whisk together rice vinegar, sesame oil, pepper, and garlic.
8. Transfer the broccoli, nuts, and raisins to the rice vinegar dressing.
9. Serve and enjoy.

# Quinoa Lentil Salad

Ingredients:
- 2/3 cups dried brown lentils
- 2 cups water
- 1 cup quinoa
- 1 yellow sweet pepper, diced
- 1 shallot, chopped
- 1 bunch arugula, finely chopped
- 2 tsp. Dijon mustard
- 1/4 cup lemon juice
- 1/4 cup extra virgin olive oil
- 1/3 cup crumbled feta cheese
- 1 pinch salt
- 4 tbsp. fresh mint, chopped

Instructions:
1. Bring 2 cups of salt water to a boil in a saucepan.
2. Toss veggies into boiling salt water. Lower heat, and cook for 30 minutes.
3. Drain lentils and discard water. Set veggies aside.
4. Boil another batch of saltwater, and cook the quinoa in the pan.
5. In a bowl, mix pepper, salt, mustard, lemon juice, and oil.
6. Place veggies in a larger bowl, and pour the mixture.
7. Sprinkle mint and feta cheese over the salad.
8. Serve and enjoy

# Spinach and Watercress Salad

Ingredients:
- 1 cup watercress, washed with stems removed
- 3 cups baby spinach, washed with stems removed
- 1 medium sliced avocado
- 1/4 cup avocado oil
- 1/8 cup lemon juice
- a pinch of salt

Instructions:
1. Pat dry the spinach and watercress. Remove the stem and separate the leaves.
2. On a large serving plate, combine the leaves of the watercress and the spinach.
3. Cut the avocado in half, then remove the pit. Peel the skin off from each side.
4. Slice the avocados into thin strips. Set aside.
5. Prepare the dressing by combining avocado oil and lemon juice.
6. Arrange the avocado strips on top of the watercress and spinach.
7. Season with salt and pepper.

# Avocado and Quinoa Salad

Ingredients:
- 4 avocados cut into pieces
- 1 cup of quinoa
- 400 grams of chickpeas
- 30 grams of fresh parsley

Instructions:
1. In a pot, boil quinoa with 2 cups of water.
2. Reduce heat to a simmer, cover, and cook for 12 minutes until water is evaporated.
3. Fluff with a fork until grains are swollen and glassy.
4. Toss all the ingredients together.
5. Season with sea salt and black pepper.
6. Serve warm with lemon wedges and olive oil.

# Spinach Salad Mix

Ingredients:
- 1 cup mushrooms, sliced thickly
- 2/3 cup olive oil
- 1 cup apple cider vinegar
- oregano
- salt
- 1 cup fresh spinach, stems trimmed
- freshly ground black pepper
- guacamole

Instructions:
1. Combine spinach and mushrooms in a large mixing bowl. Whisk together the olive oil, vinegar, oregano, and a little salt.
2. Pour the dressing over the salad and toss gently until every leaf is evenly coated.
3. Grind some black pepper over the salad and toss it again lightly.
4. Upon serving, divide the salad among bowls. Garnish with guacamole.

# Salmon Salad

Ingredients:
- 2 large filets of wild salmon, either poached or grilled and then chilled
- 1 cup cherry tomatoes, halved
- 2 red onions, sliced
- 1 tbsp. balsamic vinegar
- 1 tbsp. capers
- 1 tbsp. fresh dill, finely chopped
- 1 tbsp. extra-virgin olive oil
- 1/4 tsp. pepper, freshly ground
- salt

Instructions:
1. Remove skin and bones from the cooled salmon.
2. Break salmon into chunks, and place them into a bowl.
3. Add tomatoes, red onion, and capers. Toss ingredients.
4. Combine balsamic vinegar, olive oil, and dill in a separate bowl.
5. Pour the mixture over the salmon chunks. Toss again.
6. Sprinkle it with salt and pepper to taste.
7. Chill salad for at least half an hour before serving.

# Savory Chicken and Lentil Soup

Ingredients:
- 12 oz. or about 3 pcs. chicken thighs, remove bones, skin, and fat
- 1 lb. dried lentils
- 8 cups water
- 1/4 cup cilantro, chopped or minced
- 3 cloves garlic, minced
- 2 scallions, minced
- 1 ripe tomato, minced
- 1 onion, minced
- 1 tbsp. chicken stock
- 1 tsp. cumin
- 1 tsp. garlic powder
- 1/4 tsp. oregano
- 1/4 tsp. Spanish paprika, ground annatto seed, or Sazon seasoning
- salt

Instructions:
1. Place chicken thighs, lentils, water, and chicken stock in a large pot.
2. Cover the pot before boiling using medium-low heat for about 20 minutes, or until the chicken thighs are cooked through.
3. Take out chicken thighs from the pot to shred them.
4. Return shredded chicken to the pot.

5. Add other ingredients, except salt, into the pot.

6. Boil for about 25 minutes, or until the lentils are cooked.

7. Pour more water if the soup has thickened too much.

8. Season with salt according to your taste.

9. Enjoy it while it's hot.

# Chicken and Broccoli Casserole

Ingredients:
- 1 tbsp. olive oil
- 1/2 red onion, diced
- 1 tbsp. garlic, minced
- 1 cup uncooked brown rice
- 1 tsp. rosemary
- 1 tsp. thyme
- 1 lb. chicken breast, chopped into 1-inch pieces
- 3-1/2 cups low sodium chicken broth
- 1/2 cup (4 oz.) 2% Greek yogurt
- 2/3 cup 3-cheese blend
- 12 oz. raw broccoli florets

Instructions:
1. Set the slow cooker to low heat sauté function
2. Sauté olive oil, garlic, and onion until the onions caramelize.
3. Add uncooked brown rice, fresh rosemary, and fresh thyme.
4. Mix well. Ensure that every grain of rice is covered in the seasoning.
5. Add in chicken broth, followed by raw chicken breasts. Stir.
6. Pop the top of the slow cooker. Adjust to medium-high heat and cook for 3 to 5 hours.
7. An hour before the cooking time ends, mix it again.

8. Put in cheese and Greek yogurt. Mix it until creamy.

9. Add florets on top of the rice.

10. Season to taste with sea salt and pepper.

# Sesame Chicken

Ingredients:
Coating & Chicken:
- 1 egg
- 1 lb. chicken thighs, cut into bite-sized pieces
- 1 tbsp. arrowroot powder
- 1 tbsp. toasted sesame seed oil
- salt
- pepper

Sesame Sauce:
- 1 tbsp. toasted sesame seed oil
- 1 tbsp. vinegar
- 2 tbsp. soy sauce
- ginger, cubed into 1 cm
- 2 tbsp. Sukrin Gold
- 2 tbsp. sesame seeds
- 1/4 tsp. xanthan gum
- 1 clove garlic

Instructions:
1. Combine and whisk well egg and arrowroot powder.
2. Place chicken thigh pieces in.
3. In a large frying pan, heat up sesame seed oil.
4. Cook the chicken pieces. Make sure there are gaps between the meat.
5. In a bowl, combine and whisk all the ingredients for the sauce.

6. After cooking all the chicken pieces, pour in the sesame sauce to the pan. Stir and cook for about 5 more minutes, or until the sauce thickens.

7. Transfer chicken on top of cooked broccoli.

8. Upon serving, sprinkle with green onion and sesame seeds.

# Grilled Lamb

Ingredients:
- 1-1/2 lb. baby spinach leaves
- 3 tbsp. dried oregano, chopped
- 1/4 cup lemon juice
- 1/4 cup olive oil
- 2 tbsp. ground cumin
- 1 tsp. crushed red pepper
- 1 tbsp. coarse sea salt
- 1 tbsp. squeezed juice from an orange
- 3 cloves garlic
- 2 yellow onions, chopped
- cooking spray

Instructions:
1. In a 2-gallon zip bag, put the lamb together with the lemon juice, oregano, cumin, and salt.
2. Close the bag and refrigerate overnight
3. Puree onions, garlic, some orange juice, and olive oil in a blender.
4. Transfer to a small bowl with a cover.
5. Chill overnight.
6. Mix sea salt, red pepper, and cumin in a small bowl
7. Remove refrigerated lamb and let it sit for 30 minutes.
8. Preheat the grill to medium.
9. Place lamb on the grill and coat with some cooking spray or oil.

10. Grill lamb for one and a half hours over medium heat.
11. Remove the lamb from the grill.
12. Serve hot.

## **Baked Chicken Breasts**

Ingredients:
For the chicken breast:
- 4 chicken breasts, boneless and skinless
- 1 tbsp. olive oil
- 4 cups lukewarm water

For the chicken seasoning blend:
- 1/2 tsp. paprika, sweet or smoked
- 1/4 tsp. salt
- 1/4 tsp. fresh ground pepper
- 1/2 tsp. garlic powder
- 1/8 tsp. pepper
- 1/2 tsp. onion powder
- 1/2 tsp. dried thyme
- 1/2 tsp. dried rosemary
- 1/4 tsp. parsley, dried or fresh, chopped, for garnish

Instructions:
1. Preheat the oven to 425℉.
2. Combine lukewarm water and salt in a large bowl.
3. Add the chicken breasts. Leave for 20 to 30 minutes.
4. In a separate container, combine the dry ingredients of the seasoning blend with a fork.
5. Pour out the salt water. Rinse each chicken breast under cold water. Dry.

6. Place the chicken in a baking dish and rub olive oil all over.

7. Evenly apply seasoning blend over the chicken on all sides.

8. Place in the oven to cook for 22 to 25 minutes. Check if the internal temperature reaches 165°F.

9. Make sure to keep an eye on the breasts, as each piece may cook faster than the rest.

10. Broil the chicken until the top parts are golden.

11. If you want a browned and crispier top, set the oven to broil on high for the final 4 minutes.

12. Transfer to a serving plate to rest for 10 minutes before cutting.

13. Garnish with parsley upon serving.

# Ginger Chicken Stir Fry

Ingredients:
Stir-fry mix:
- 1 lb. cooked chicken, dark or light meat
- 4 cups cremini mushrooms, sliced
- 4 cups purple cabbage, sliced
- 2 cups carrots
- 1/2 cup green onions, cut slanted
- 3 cups cauliflower florets
- 1 handful enoki mushrooms
- 2 tbsp. avocado oil
- 1 package rice noodles, cook according to instructions

Stir-fry sauce:
- 4 cloves minced garlic
- 1/4 cup honey
- 1/4 tsp. grated ginger
- 1/4 cup rice wine vinegar
- 1 tsp. favorite hot sauce
- 1 cup chicken stock
- 1 tbsp. avocado oil

Instructions:
To make the stir-fry sauce:
1. Cook garlic with oil on low to medium heat
2. Once the garlic is browned, add in the honey. Let the sauce bubble for a moment.

3. Add in the vinegar and cover with a lid.

4. Pour in the chicken stock. Leave to boil until reduced by half.

5. Season with salt and pepper. Add your favorite hot sauce.

To make the stir-fry mix:

1. Heat the oil in a large wok. Cook the vegetables, adding one-by-one according to the degree of hardness.

2. Once the vegetables are well-caramelized, add in the chicken and noodles and heat through.

3. Pour in the stir-fry sauce and mix well.

4. Garnish with green onions

# Baked Salmon with Dill and Lemon

Ingredients:
- 1-1/4 lb. salmon—king, sockeye, or coho salmon
- 1/4 tsp. black pepper, to taste
- 3 cloves garlic, minced or 1 tsp. garlic powder
- 1 tbsp. fresh chopped dill
- 2 tbsp. olive oil
- 1 tbsp. lemon juice

Instructions:
1. Preheat the oven to 350oF.
2. Grease a sheet pan with olive oil.
3. Season salmon on both sides with salt and pepper.
4. Combine olive oil, lemon juice, dill, and garlic in a small container.
5. In the baking dish, place the salmon skin-side down.
6. Drizzle the mixture over the fish and spread evenly on top.
7. Bake the salmon until the top is not opaque anymore, about 15-20 minutes.
8. To get a golden brown color on top, broil the fish at 425oF for a minute. Watch over it and check the middle temperature until it reaches 145oF.
9. Upon serving, garnish the salmon with dill and lemon slices.

# Pepitas-Kale Soup

Ingredients:
- 1/2 cup raw pepitas
- 2-1/2 cups water
- 3 cups kale, chopped
- 1/4 cup apple juice
- 3 tbsp. lemon juice
- 1 tbsp. fresh ginger, minced
- 1 tsp. hot pepper, diced
- 1/2 cup avocado, mashed
- 1/8 tsp. ground black pepper
- 1-1/2 tsp. salt
- 1 tbsp. cilantro, minced
- a pinch of cayenne pepper
- 1/4 cup red bell pepper, minced

Instructions:
1. Soak pepitas in water for a few minutes. Drain and rinse.
2. Place inside the blender together with all the ingredients except for the cilantro and bell pepper.
3. Blend until it becomes creamy.
4. Place all in a separate bowl.
5. Add cilantro then stir well.
6. Top red bell peppers upon serving.

# Broccoli Soup

Ingredients:
- 1 onion, chopped
- 1 lb. broccoli, chopped
- 1 small tomato, chopped
- 1 tbsp. grapeseed oil
- 1/2 cup unsweetened almond milk
- 16 oz. water
- 1/4 tsp. turmeric
- cayenne pepper, to taste

Instructions:
1. Put oil and onion in a medium pot. Saute over medium heat for about a couple of minutes.
2. Add the seasoning, tomato, and broccoli. Saute for 10 more minutes.
3. Add 6 ounces of water. Cover the pot and let it simmer for a couple more minutes.
4. Transfer the contents into a blender, followed by the remaining water and milk. Blend for a couple of minutes.
5. Pour back the blended ingredients into the pot.
6. Raise up the heat and boil for a couple of minutes.
7. Serve and enjoy while hot.

# Udon Salmon Soup

Ingredients:
- 8 oz. dried udon noodles, may also use ramen or soba, cooked and drained according to package instructions
- 1 clove garlic, smashed and peeled
- 4 oz. cremini mushrooms or button mushrooms, sliced thinly
- 2 scallions, sliced thinly
- 8 oz. salmon fillet, skinned and cut into 1-inch cubes
- 2 tbsp. white miso
- 1 cup boiling water
- 2 cups chicken or vegetable broth, homemade or store-bought, no salt added
- 1/2 tsp. seasoned rice vinegar
- 1 tsp. oyster sauce
- 1/4 tsp. toasted sesame oil

Instructions:
1. Boil a kettle of water.
2. Dissolve the miso in a cup of boiling water.
3. Pour the mixture through a fine-mesh strainer into a heavy saucepan or Dutch oven over medium heat.
4. Add broth, garlic, oyster sauce, and rice vinegar.
5. Once the mixture starts bubbling, reduce the heat to medium-low and cook for 5 minutes.

6. Stir in mushrooms and salmon. Cook for 15 minutes.

7. Remove the saucepan from the heat and stir in scallion, toasted sesame oil, and cooked udon noodles. Discard garlic.

8. Let sit for 3 to 5 minutes before serving.

# Lentil Soup

Ingredients:
- 1 tbsp. avocado oil
- 1 cup onion, diced
- 1/2 cup carrot, diced
- 1/2 cup celery, diced
- 4 cups vegetable or chicken broth
- 1 cup dried red lentils, well rinsed
- 1/4 tsp dried thyme
- 1/2 cup fresh flat-leaf parsley, chopped
- salt
- pepper

Instructions:
1. Sauté carrot, celery, and onion in a large saucepan over medium heat. Do so until they are soft.
2. Pour in the broth with lentils and thyme and wait to boil.
3. Lower the heat. Cover and leave to simmer until lentils are soft, about 20 minutes.
4. Transfer the soup to a blender.
5. Set the blender on high. Purée the soup until it's creamy.
6. If it's too thick, pour in a cup of water.
7. Add salt and pepper to taste.
8. Return to the saucepan to reheat if necessary.
9. Ladle into bowls and garnish with parsley.
10. Serve and enjoy while hot.

# Instant Pot Bone Broth

Ingredients:
- 1 instant pot
- 4 whole celeries, ribbed
- 3 whole carrots, halved
- 1 onion, sliced in half
- 3 to 4 lb. beef bones, preferably grass-fed, roasted
- 1 bay leaf
- 2 cloves garlic, crushed with a knife
- 1 tbsp. apple cider vinegar
- 1 tsp. Himalayan pink salt

Instructions:
1. Put the beef bones on a baking sheet made of glass and season as desired with a sprinkle of salt.
2. Place the bones in an oven preheated to 420°F and let them roast for 30 minutes.
3. Flip them over and leave them for another 20 minutes.
4. Place the ingredients in the instant pot. Add the bones first, then followed by the remaining vegetables and seasoning.
5. Pour in clean water until it reaches an inch below the instant pot's max fill line.
6. Seal the instant pot and leave it on manual high pressure for approximately 75 minutes.
7. Remove both the vegetables and bones and filter the broth using a fine-mesh strainer.

8. Pour the broth back into the instant pot.
9. You may use it immediately as a soup base or let it cool before storing it in the freezer for future use.

# **Macrobiotic Bowl Medley**

Ingredients:
- 1/2 cup brown rice
- 3 cup chard, roughly chopped
- 1 cup squash, diced
- 1 cup broccoli florets
- 1 cup black beans, thoroughly rinsed and drained
- 1 oz. kombu
- 1/2 cup sauerkraut, chopped

Sauce:
- 2 tbsp. sesame tahini
- 2 tbsp. sodium tamari
- 1 clove garlic
- 1 tbsp. ginger
- 1 lime, juiced

Instructions:
1. Boil 1 cup of water.
2. Add rice and allow it to boil. Cover and reduce heat and simmer for 40 minutes.
3. Remove from heat and allow to sit covered for another 10 minutes, then fluff with a fork.
4. Place beans in a pot with kombu. Cover with water, and bring to a boil.
5. Reduce heat and simmer for 15-20 minutes. Drain and rinse after.

6. Place a steamer basket in a pot with water and bring it to a boil.

7. Add broccoli, cover, and steam for 4-5 minutes then remove, keeping water in the pot.

8. Add squash, cover, and steam for 4-5 minutes then remove, keeping water in the pot.

9. Add chard, cover, and steam for 3-4 minutes, then remove.

10. Mix all the ingredients of the sauce.

11. Serve everything on a plate and enjoy!

## Conclusion

There is no treatment available for the MTHFR mutations as they don't require it. It is, however, highly recommended that people who experience these undergo lifestyle changes such as keeping healthy and changing their diet, particularly good sources of folic acid, vitamin B12, riboflavin, and vitamin C, to name a few. Doing so somehow offsets the deficiency.

By simply following the list of food items that you need to include and remove from your diet, you're giving yourself a chance to feel better. Not only that, following a healthier diet and lifestyle will also be beneficial for you in the long run.

Following a healthier lifestyle may seem like a simple solution for health problems that seem complex, but it does work. It may be challenging at first, but if it helps you in the long run, then it wouldn't hurt to try. Similar to any diet program, it's highly recommended that you consult with your doctor first if following the MTHFR diet will be beneficial for you.

Thank you again for getting this guide.

If you found this guide helpful, please take the time to share your thoughts and post a review. It'd be greatly appreciated!

# Thank you and good luck!

# References

A balanced approach to the 'MTHFR diet.' (2021, March 24). https://drruscio.com/mthfr-diet/.

CDC. (2022, June 15). Mthfr gene and folic acid. Centers for Disease Control and Prevention. https://www.cdc.gov/ncbddd/folicacid/mthfr-gene-and-folic-acid.html.

Chung, Y. J., Robert, C., Gough, S. M., Rassool, F. V., & Aplan, P. D. (2014). Oxidative stress leads to increased mutation frequency in a murine model of myelodysplastic syndrome. Leukemia Research, 38(1), 95–102. https://doi.org/10.1016/j.leukres.2013.07.008.

Folate, MTHFR gene and heart health. (n.d.). Retrieved December 17, 2022, from https://www.gbhealthwatch.com/GND-Cardiovascular-Diseases-MTHFR.php.

Good foods for MTHFR: What to eat • MTHFR living. (2013, July 28). MTHFR Living. https://mthfrliving.com/food-and-recipes/ingredients/good-foods-mthfr-what-to-eat/.

Graydon, J. S., Claudio, K., Baker, S., Kocherla, M., Ferreira, M., Roche-Lima, A., Rodríguez-Maldonado, J., Duconge, J., & Ruaño, G. (2019). Ethnogeographic prevalence and implications of the 677C>T and 1298A>C MTHFR polymorphisms in US primary care populations. Biomarkers in Medicine, 13(8), 649–661. https://doi.org/10.2217/bmm-2018-0392.

Leaky gut, MTHFR, and how to fix it—Doctor Doni. (2017, October 19). https://doctordoni.com/2017/10/leaky-gut-mthfr-and-how-to-fix-it/.

Lum, A. & Perishable. (2020, August 18). What you need to eat (And avoid!) for MTHFR. MTHFR Support Australia. https://mthfrsupport.com.au/2020/08/what-you-need-to-eat-and-avoid-for-mthfr/.

Moll, S., & Varga, E. A. (2015). Homocysteine and MTHFR Mutations. Circulation, 132(1). https://doi.org/10.1161/CIRCULATIONAHA.114.013311.

MTHFR gene: Medlineplus genetics. (n.d.). Retrieved December 17, 2022, from https://medlineplus.gov/genetics/gene/mthfr/.

Nutrition, C. F., MPH in. (2022, April 12). Best MTHFR diet, lifestyle, & supplements. Clean Eating Kitchen.

https://www.cleaneatingkitchen.com/mthfr-diet-lifestyle-supplements/.

Restorative wellness center—Blog. (n.d.). Restorative Wellness Center. Retrieved December 17, 2022, from https://www.restorativechiro.com/blog/2019/10/27/diet-considerations-for-those-with-mthfr.

The MTHFR diet? Don't waste your time. (2020, December 7). Gene Food. https://www.mygenefood.com/blog/why-an-mthfr-eating-plan-isnt-necessary/.

Toxins and heavy metals: How they affect MTHFR and methylation and 7 tips to avoid them - Doctor Doni. (2017, September 28). https://doctordoni.com/2017/09/toxins-and-heavy-metals/.

Printed in the USA
CPSIA information can be obtained
at www.ICGtesting.com
LVHW020719011124
795404LV00053B/704

9 781088 091913